C000041948

The Complete Keto Diet CookBook For Women Over 50

Low-Carb High-Fat Recipes for your Keto Day

Rose Pope

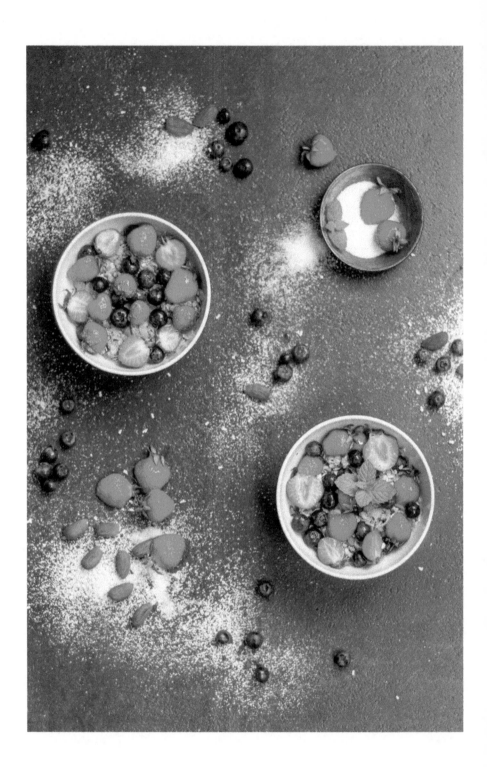

© Copyright 2021 - All rights reserved.

The content contained within this book may not be reproduced, duplicated or transmitted without direct written permission from the author or the publisher.

Under no circumstances will any blame or legal responsibility be held against the publisher, or author, for any damages, reparation, or monetary loss due to the information contained within this book. Either directly or indirectly.

Legal Notice:

This book is copyright protected. This book is only for personal use. You cannot amend, distribute, sell, use, quote or paraphrase any part, or the content within this book, without the consent of the author or publisher.

Disclaimer Notice:

Please note the information contained within this document is for educational and entertainment purposes only. All effort has been executed to present accurate, up to date, and reliable, complete information. No warranties of any kind are declared or implied. Readers acknowledge that the author is not engaging in the rendering of legal, financial, medical or professional advice. The content within this book has been derived from various sources. Please consult a licensed professional before attempting any techniques outlined in this book.

By reading this document, the reader agrees that under no circumstances is the author responsible for any losses, direct or indirect, which are incurred as a result of the use of information contained within this document, including, but not limited to, — errors, omissions, or inaccuracies.

Table of Contents

Main Dish

Breakfast

1   Cod Scrambled Eggs

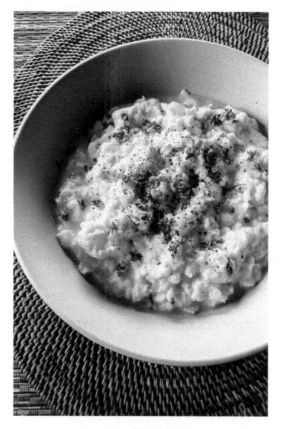

Servings: 2 | **Time:** 30 mins | **Difficulty:** Easy

Nutrients per serving: Calories: 286 kcal | Fat: 17g | Carbohydrates: 3.9g | Protein: 28.1g | Fiber: 0.4g

Ingredients

1 Tbsp. Olive Oil

4 Eggs

1/4 Tsp. Sea Salt

1/2 Tbsp. Water

1/2 Cup Leeks, Sliced Thinly

Salt, To Taste

1 Cod Fillet, Fresh

Method

1.   Take cold water in a bowl and put the sliced leeks in it. Cover it and set aside.

2.   Season the cod fillet with salt after drying. Heat 1 tsp oil in a skillet over medium-high flame and fry the fish in it for 2-3 minutes on each side until become golden. Reduce the flame to medium-low and break the fish with the spoon into pieces.

3.   Drain the leeks, pat dry them. Add 1/2 tsp more oil in the pan, heat it and cook the leeks in it with fish for about 2-3 minutes until become soft.

4.   Take the pan off the stove and let cool for a few minutes.

5. Combine eggs and water in a bowl and whisk until become frothy.

6. Place the pan back on the stove, add the remaining oil in it and heat it over low flame.

7. Pour the eggs in the pan, let them set for a while, then scramble them. Sprinkle salt over the cod scramble eggs, mix to combine, and take off the stove once done.

2   Instant Pot Breakfast Casserole With Sausage

Servings: 6 | **Time**: 40 mins | **Difficulty**: Easy

Nutrients per serving: Calories: 327 kcal | Fat: 22.8g | Carbohydrates: 0.4g | Protein: 26.7g

Ingredients

4 Eggs

2/3 Cup Cheddar Cheese, Grated

2/3 Cup Chicken Broth

2 Cups Italian Sausage, Ground

Cooking Spray

Method

1.   Set sauté mode on Instant Pot and sauté the ground sausage in it until cooked thoroughly.

2.   Combine all the ingredients in a bowl and whisk well. Add in the sausage as well, once cooked.

3.   Spray a cake pan with cooking oil spray and pour the mixture in it.

4.   Pour one cup water in a trivet and put it in the Instant Pot. Put the cake pan in the Instant Pot and seal it.

5.   Cook for about 28 minutes or until the eggs are cooked.

6.   Wait for 10 minutes before opening the Instant Pot.

3   Low Carb Quiche With Almond Flour Crust

Servings: 8 | **Time**: 1 hr. 10 mins | **Difficulty**: Easy

Nutrients per serving: Calories: 311 kcal | Fat: 24.8g | Carbohydrates: 11.8g | Protein: 12.5g | Fiber: 2.5g

Ingredients

1 Cup Pork, Ground

1/2 Tsp. Sea Salt

1/8 Tsp. Paprika Powder

1 Pie Crust, Low Carb

1/8 Tsp. Fennel Seed

1/4 Tsp. Salt

1/2 Tsp. Parsley, Dried

1/4 Tsp. Red Pepper Flakes

1/2 Cup Coconut Milk

1/2 Tsp. Italian Seasoning

1/4 Tsp. Onion Powder

1/4 + 1/8 Tsp. Black Pepper, Ground

5 Eggs

1 Cup Spinach, Chopped

Method

1.   Preheat the oven to 375 degrees F.

2.   Brown the ground pork in a skillet over medium heat with all the spices. Remove from heat once done.

3.   Combine the eggs with coconut milk spinach, cooked pork, and salt in a bowl and whisk well.

4.   Pour the mixture in the pie crust and put in the preheated oven.

5.   Bake for 20 minutes, take out and cover with foil, put back and bake for another 18-20 minutes or until the quiche is cooked.

4   Keto Low Carb Egg Wraps

Servings: 2 | **Time:** 15 mins | **Difficulty:** Easy

Nutrients per serving: Calories: 240 kcal | Fat: 18g | Carbohydrates: 6g | Protein: 14g | Fiber: 3g

Ingredients

1/2 Tomato, Sliced

2 Bacon Strips, Cooked

Salt, To Taste

2 Eggs

1/2 Avocado, Sliced

Black Pepper, To Taste

1 Tbsp. Almond Milk

Cooking Spray

1/4 Cup Cheddar Cheese, Grated (Optional)

Method

1.   Spray a pan with cooking spray and heat it over low flame.

2.   Whisk the eggs with salt and pepper in a bowl and pour 1/4 cup of this mixture into the pan. Swirl the pan to spread he mixture in the pan evenly.

3.   Cover the pan and let it cook for a few minutes, then flip and cook on the other side, until becomes golden.

4.   Similarly make another egg tortilla with the remaining egg mixture.

5.   Place the egg tortillas on serving plates, put one bacon strip on each and top with sliced tomatoes and avocados.

6.   Sprinkle with grated cheese on top.

5   Savory Egg Custard

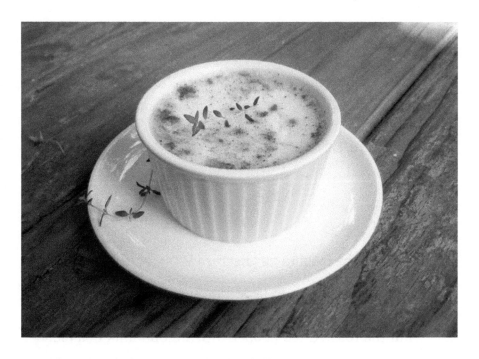

Servings: 4 | **Time**: 50 mins | **Difficulty:** Easy

Nutrients per serving: Calories: 240 kcal | Fat: 18g | Carbohydrates: 6g | Protein: 14g | Fiber: 3g

Ingredients

1/4 Cup Greek Yogurt, Plain

3 Eggs

1 Tbsp. Water

1/4 Tsp. Salt

1 Cup Almond Milk, Unsweetened

1/2 Tsp. Garlic Powder

1 Red Pepper, Roasted

Cooking Spray

Goat Cheese, To Taste

Method

1.   Preheat the oven to 325 degrees F.

2.   Take 4 ramekins and grease them with cooking spray.

3.   Put the roasted red pepper with almond milk in a blender and blend until become smooth. Strain it for any chunks and put in the blender again.

4.   Add all the other ingredients in it too except for goat cheese.

5.   Blend until a smooth mixture is formed.

6.   Divide this mixture into 4 ramekins and put them in the preheated oven.

7.   Bake for 35-40 minutes or until cooked through.

8.   Let cool for an hour and then garnish with goat cheese.

Lunch

6 Roasted Butternut Squash Soup With Sausage

Servings: 12 | **Time:** 1 hr 15 mins | **Difficulty**: Easy

Nutrients per serving: Calories: 272 kcal | Fat: 22.4g | Carbohydrates: 8.8g | Protein: 9.2g | Fiber: 1.4g

Ingredients

¼ Tsp. nutmeg

½ Tsp. ground ginger

1 ½ Tsps. rubbed sage

1 cup heavy cream

1 large butternut squash (about 4 pounds), peeled and cubed

1 medium onion, chopped

1 pound ground sausage

1 Tsp. sea salt

2 Tbsps. olive oil

3 Tbsps. butter or olive oil

4 cups chicken stock, divided

6 cloves garlic, minced

fried sage leaves, optional garnish

Pinch of cayenne pepper

roasted pepitas, optional garnish

Sea salt and ground black pepper

sour cream, optional garnish

Method

1. Layer the squash on a baking sheet.

2. Season with pepper and salt and drizzle with olive oil.

3. Roast for 40 minutes at 375°F.

4. Melt the butter in a Dutch oven.

5. Add the ginger, garlic, onion, salt, cayenne, sage, and nutmeg.

6. Blend the onion mixture.

7. Blend the roasted squash, the onions the chicken stock.

8. Cook the sausage on medium heat.

9. Put the pureed squash with the sausage.

10. Cook on medium heat for 10 minutes, stirring frequently,

11. Then reduce heat to low and let simmer for 30 minutes.

12. Top with fried sage, pepitas, and sour cream.

13. Serve.

7   Reuben Stuffed Mushrooms

Servings: 5 | **Time**: 30 mins | **Difficulty:** Easy

Nutrients per serving: Calories: 190 kcal | Fat: 20g | Carbohydrates: 1.5g | Protein: 0g | Fiber: 0g

Ingredients

¼ cup Keto Russian Dressing, more to taste

½ cup sauerkraut, chopped

½ cup shredded Swiss cheese, or 5 slices

1 Tbsp. chopped fresh chives

5 large portobello mushrooms, cleaned, with gills and stems removed

8 ounces corned beef, sliced or chopped

cracked black pepper, to taste Russian Dressing

½ cup ketchup

1 cup mayonnaise

1 Tbsp. chopped fresh chives

1 Tbsp. chopped fresh parsley

1 Tbsp. Worcestershire sauce

1 Tsp. chopped fresh dill

2 Tbsps. spicy brown mustard

Method

1.   In a large bowl, Mix ketchup, mayonnaise, Worcestershire sauce, mustard, chives, parsley, and dill to make Russian Dressing.

2.   In a mixing bowl, combine the corned beef, sauerkraut, and Russian dressing.

3.   Put mixture in each cap of mushroom and add swiss cheese on top of it.

4.   Bake them at 400°F for 15 minutes.

5.   Top with black pepper and chives.

6.   Serve.

8   Reuben Stuffed Sweet Potatoes With Russian Dressing

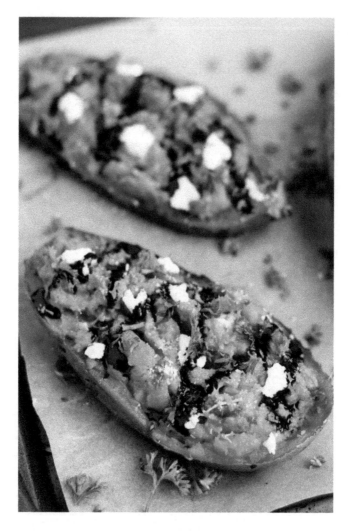

Servings: 6 | **Time**: 25 mins | **Difficulty**: Easy

Nutrients per serving: Calories: 660 kcal | Fat: 60g | Carbohydrates: 7g | Protein: 13g | Fiber: 7g

Ingredients

FOR THE REUBEN STUFFED SWEET POTATOES

¼ cup butter (½ stick)

⅓ cup Russian Dressing

1 lb precooked deli style corned beef, chopped

1 tsp caraway seeds

1 tsp onion powder

1½ cups sauerkraut

2 large sweet potatoes

2 tbsp olive oil

3 cloves garlic, minced

4 slices Swiss cheese

Chopped green onion, for garnish

FOR THE RUSSIAN DRESSING

½ cup ketchup (reduced sugar, organic preferred)

1 cup mayonnaise

1 tbsp fresh chives, chopped

1 tbsp fresh parsley, chopped

1 tbsp Worcestershire sauce

1 tsp fresh dill, chopped

2 tbsp spicy brown mustard

Method

FOR THE REUBEN STUFFED SWEET POTATOES

1.   Put butter on sweet potato.

2.   Sprinkle with the caraway seeds and onion powder. Bake them for 45 minutes to 1 hour.

3.   Add the sauerkraut, corned beef, and garlic in heated olive oil.

4.   Sauté for 10 minutes.

5.   Put corned beef mixture on top of sweet potato baked.

6.   Add a slice of Swiss cheese on top and drizzle with Russian dressing.

FOR THE RUSSIAN DRESSING

1.   In a large mixing bowl, mix ketchup, mayonnaise, chives, parsley, mustard, Worcestershire sauce, and dill.

2.   Mix well. Serve

9   One Pot Keto Sesame Chicken And Broccoli

Servings: 4 | **Time:** 25 mins | **Difficulty:** Easy

Nutrients per serving: Calories: 204 kcal | Fat: 6.1g | Carbohydrates: 7g | Protein: 30g | Fiber: 2.1g

Ingredients

¼ cup coconut aminos, or soy sauce

½ Tsp. sesame seeds, plus extra for garnish

1 ½ Tsp. arrowroot powder (get it here)

1 clove garlic, minced

1 pound boneless, skinless chicken breast, cubed

1 Tbsp. avocado oil (I use this brand)

1 Tsp. sesame oil

12 ounces broccoli florets

Green onions, sliced, for garnish

Red pepper flakes, for garnish

Salt and pepper, to taste

Method

1.   Microwave the broccoli florets with some water to tender it.

2.   Mix the arrowroot powder and coconut aminos in a small bowl.

3.   Add the garlic and avocado oil and sauté until fragrant in a large skillet.

4.   Sauté the chicken with pepper and salt to taste in a skillet.

5.   Sauté the broccoli and sesame oil in a pan then put coconut amino mixture on top of it.

6.   Garnish with sesame seeds, red pepper flakes, and green onions.

7.   Serve.

10   Cabbage Noodle Tuna Casserole

Servings: 8 | **Time:** 45 mins | **Difficulty:** Easy

Nutrients per serving: Calories: 377 kcal | Fat: 28g | Carbohydrates: 10g | Protein: 23.5g | Fiber: 3g

Ingredients

½ cup frozen peas

1 ¼ cup Parmesan cheese, grated, divided

1 ½ cup heavy cream

1 cup onion, chopped

2 cloves garlic, minced

2 tbsp grass-fed butter

2 tbsp lemon zest

2 tbsp olive oil

2 tsp dried dill or

2 tbsp fresh dill

2 tsp dry mustard powder (get it here)

3- 5oz cans albacore tuna, drained (I use this brand)

3 ribs celery, chopped

juice of 1 lemon

medium head green cabbage (about 1 ½ lbs), cut into large shreds

sea salt and black pepper, to taste

Method

1.   Heat the butter and olive oil in skillet.

2.   Once heated, add the onion, cabbage, garlic, celery, black pepper, and sea salt to the pan.

3.   Sauté to crisp the vegetables for about 10 minutes.

4.   Mix in the mustard powder, dill, lemon juice, and lemon zest.

5.   Pour the 1 cup Parmesan cheese and heavy cream into the pan.

6.   Melt cheese while stirring.

7.   Decrease heat and let the sauce to thicken.

8.   Stir in the peas and the tuna.

9.   Drizzle Parmesan cheese over the dish and put it in the oven. Cook until the cheese top is golden brown.

Dinner

11   Tandoori Shrimp

Servings: 4 | **Time:** 30 mins | **Difficulty**: Easy

Nutrients per serving: Calories: 247 kcal | Fat: 9g | Carbohydrates: 7g | Protein: 36g | Fiber: 3g

Ingredients

Half cup of coconut milk (full-fat) or coconut yogurt (plain)

1 and a half pounds of shrimp (21 to 25 shrimps) peeled & deveined

¼ cup roughly chopped fresh cilantro

1 tbsp. of spice tandoori mix (make sure no salt is added)

1 tbsp. of freshly squeezed lemon juice

2 limes, slice into thin wedges

Half tsp. of Crystal Diamond kosher salt

Method

1.   Thaw the shrimps, if they are frozen in running water for 6 to 7 minutes, or until they thaw slightly. Clean the shrimps if they have not been cleaned before.

2.   In a mixing bowl, add coconut milk, crystal Diamond kosher salt, freshly squeezed lemon juice, and spice Tandoori mix. Mix well and set it aside. If using shake up bottle, shake and take out a half cup of marinade.

3.   Toss the cleaned shrimps in marinade well. Keep the marinated shrimps in the fridge for half an hour.

4.   Let the oven preheat to 400 F with the middle rack.

5.   Place the marinated shrimps in one even layer on the parchment-lined baking rimmed sheet.

6.   Roast for 7 to 8 minutes in the oven; flip the shrimps halfway through.

7.   Cooking time depends upon the size of shrimps. Even smaller shrimps will take five minutes to cook.

8.   Serve the tandoori shrimps with lime wedges and top with roughly chopped fresh cilantro and few drops of lemon juice.

9.   Serve and enjoy these delicious tandoori shrimps with rice.

12   Vietnamese Pork Stew in Instant Pot

Servings: 8 | **Time**: 1 hr 25 mins | **Difficulty:** Easy

Nutrients per serving: Calories: 500 kcal | Fat: 34g | Carbohydrates: 6g | Protein: 41g | Fiber: 2g

Ingredients

¼ cup of shallots, cut into thin slices

3 scallions cut into thin slices

1 tbsp. of avocado oil, ghee, or coconut oil

4 cloves of garlic peeled & smashed

1 cup of coconut water

¼ pound of shiitake mushrooms cut the stems & slice in half or in quarters if they are too large

3 large size peeled carrots, slice into half-inch slices (diagonal)

3 tbsp. of fish sauce and add more if needed

Half cup of fresh cilantro leaves

3 quarter size fresh slices of peeled ginger

3 pounds of pork shoulder slice into two" cubes

Method

1.   In the instant pot, turn on the function of sauteing; when the inserted metal is hot, add in the oil of your preference.

2.   Add in shiitake mushrooms, shallots. Cook for about 4 to 5 minutes or until the vegetables are tender.

3.   Add in garlic, ginger and cook for 4 to 5 minutes.

4.   Add in the meat cubes and mix it well.

5.   Add in fish sauce and coconut water.

6.   Mix well, scrape the bottom of the browned bits of the instant pot.

7.   Turn off the function of sauteing. Lock the instant pot's lids, and let it cook for 40 minutes under high pressure.

8.   As it is cooked. Let the pressure release naturally or release it manually after 15 minutes.

9.   The pork should be tender that it should be flake with a fork. If it does not flake easily, let it cook for 7 to 10 minutes more in high pressure.

10.   Taste it and add more seasoning, salt, and fish sauce if required.

11.   Keep the pork warm on a serving platter, cover it so it will remain warm.

12.   Add the carrots gently to the cooking liquid so you will not splash yourself.

13.   Let it cook for two minutes at high pressure.

14.   Release the pressure manually or naturally, then carefully remove the lid of

the instant pot.

15.   Take out the cooking liquid and carrots with the pork.

16.   Serve with scallion slices and fresh chopped cilantro and enjoy.

13   Sheet Pan Meatballs & Broccolini

Servings: 6| **Time:** 40 mins | **Difficulty:** Medium

Nutrients per serving: Calories: 531 kcal | Fat: 43g | Carbohydrates: 11g | Protein: 31g | Fiber: 3g

Ingredients

1 and a half cups of marinara sauce

2 tbsp. of avocado oil or extra virgin olive oil

1 and a half pounds of bulk Italian sausage, please ensure it is Whole30 suitable

1 pound of broccolini with trimmed ends

1 tsp. of Mushroom Magic Powder or Crystal Diamond kosher salt

Method

1.   Let the oven preheat to 400 F or 425 F convection bake, with a middle rack.

2.   Toss the broccolini with mushroom magic powder and olive oil and place on a rimmed baking sheet. Or use 1 tsp. of

crystal diamond kosher salt instead of mushroom powder or half tsp. of fine grain salt.

3.	Place the seasoned broccolini on a baking sheet in one even layer.

4.	Make some meatballs from bulk Italian sausage. Get the meat out of links by piercing it with a fork or knife.

5.	Make same size meatballs; it will make 24 meatballs that should be one and a half-inch in diameter.

6.	Place the meatballs in space available around and the broccolini on a rimmed baking sheet.

7.	Place the rimmed baking sheet in the oven. Roast the broccolini and meatballs until meatballs are cooked through or for 18 to 20 minutes.

8.	Broccolini should be charred in some places.

9.	After 7 to 10 minutes, rotate the baking tray to make sure, cooking is even.

10.	Meanwhile, in a pan, heat the marinara sauce or a microwave-safe container in a microwave.

11.	Take out the meatballs, and pour over the hot marinara sauce.

12.	Serve right away with rice and enjoy.

14   Instant Pot Orange Duck & Gravy

Servings: 4 | **Time**: 1 hr 30 mins | **Difficulty:** Easy

Nutrients per serving: Calories: 491 kcal | Fat: 27g | Carbohydrates: 11g | Protein: 49g | Fiber: 2g

Ingredients

Kosher salt (Diamond Crystal), to taste

Half tsp. of herbs de Provence

¼ tsp. of freshly cracked black pepper

4 legs' of duck

2 tbsp. of avocado oil, or ghee duck fat divided

1 yellow, medium-sized onion, chopped

1 celery rib, medium-sized, finely diced

1 carrot, large-sized, diced

8 cloves of garlic, peeled and smashed

1 tbsp. of tomato paste

Half cup of chicken stock or bone broth

1 navel orange, medium-sized

2 tbsp. of Italian parsley, roughly chopped

1 bay leaf, dried

1 sprig of thyme, fresh

Method

1.   In a mixing bowl, mix herbes de Provence, freshly cracked black pepper, one and a half tsp. of crystal diamond kosher salt.

2.   With paper towels, dry the duck's legs, and coat with the seasoning mix you prepared earlier.

3.   In the instant pot, turn the sauteed function on, and add one tbsp. of oil in it.

4.   Once the oil is hot, add diced carrots, onions, celery half tsp. of crystal diamond kosher salt. Keep stirring and cook until vegetables are tender for 3-5 minutes.

5.   Add in tomato paste and garlic. Keep stirring and cook for 30 seconds, until garlic becomes fragrant.

6.   Add in the bone broth, scrape the bottom for browned bits.

7.   Peel the orange with a peeler and add in orange zest strips, but do not peel too deeply so that the bitter part would not be peeled.

8. Squeeze the orange juice in the instant pot.

9. Add thyme, parsley, and bay leaf. Mix well, and turn the saute function off.

10. Add the duck legs (seasoned) in the instant pot, in one even layer, on vegetables. Make sure the duck is skin side up.

11. Lock the instant pot's lid, keep it in a sealed arrangement. Let it cook under high pressure for 40-45 minutes.

12. Drop the high pressure naturally of the instant pot as the duck has cooked through.

13. One can release the pressure manually after 18 to 20 minutes.

14. Take the duck legs out carefully. It should be very tender that you can break apparat with a fork, so handle it gently.

15. You can serve it right away or keep it safe in a sealed container for four days and serve as you want.

16. Take out the orange zest, sprig of thyme, bay leaf. With an immersion blender, puree the rest of the sauce to turn into a thick gravy.

17. Taste and adjust seasoning with crystal diamond kosher salt and freshly ground black pepper.

18. It will make lots of gravy, so store in the freezer in ice cube trays, and use up to four months.

19.   After patting them dry with paper towels, cook the meat in a cast-iron skillet on medium flame.

20.   Add oil to the hot cast-iron skillet. Add legs of duck, skin side down, and pan-fry them for 2 to 3 minutes, until the skin is lightly browned and crispy.

21.   Now flip the duck legs over and let them golden brown on the flip side.

22.   If you do not like the frying option. One can broil the duck legs (it will not make the skin as crispy as with frying)

23.   The broiling method: turn the broiler on, and place the duck legs on the middle rack in a rimmed baking sheet, place the skip side up.

24.   Broil the duck legs for 5 to 10 minutes until the skin is golden brown.

25.   Now serve the duck legs with thick delicious gravy. Enjoy.

15   Tandoori Fish

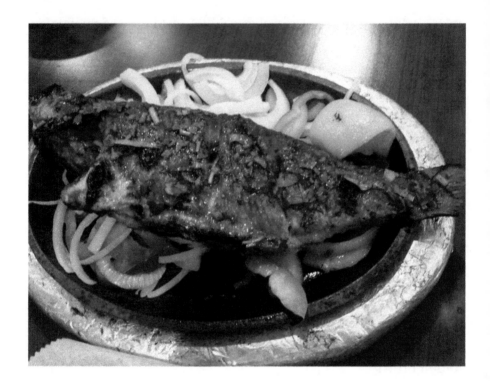

Servings: 4 | **Time:** 40 mins | **Difficulty**: Medium

Nutrients per serving: Calories: 357 kcal | Fat: 19g | Carbohydrates: 7g | Protein: 29g | Fiber: 2g

Ingredients

1 tsp. of kosher salt (Diamond Crystal) or half tsp. of a fine grain salt

4 white fish fillets (such as sea bass or cod, 6-ounce each)

1 lemon cut into thin wedges

1 tbsp. of spice tandoori mix (make sure to get no salt added)

1 tbsp. of lemon juice (freshly squeezed)

Half cup of coconut yogurt or plain coconut cream, or coconut milk (full-fat)

Method

1. With a paper towel, dab the fillets dry.

2. Season with salt on every side of fish fillets.

3. In a bowl, mix freshly squeezed lemon juice, plain yogurt, spice tandoori mix.

4. Mix well, or shake in a glass bottle and take out a half cup of marinade.

5. Coat the seasoned fish fillet in marinade well. Keep in the fridge for 20 minutes to 60 minutes. (One can skip this part and cook the fish right away).

6. Let the oven preheat to 400 F with the middle rack.

7. On a rimmed baking sheet, place a sheet of parchment paper.

8. Place all four fish fillets on them.

9.   Place the baking sheet in the oven on the middle rack and cook for 8 to 15 minutes or until the internal temperature of fish fillets shows 145 F. (cooking time depends on the thickness of fish fillet)

10.   Fish should be flaky and opaque, and it should come apart easily with the fork.

11.   As one" fish fillet takes almost ten minutes to cook and thinner fillets than that will cook faster.

12.   Serve the fish right away with sautéed vegetables and thin lemon wedges. I served mine over cauliflower rice and micro salad, vegetables.

Desserts

16 Double Chocolate Coconut Flour Muffins

Servings: 12 | **Time:** 20 mins | **Difficulty**: Easy

Nutrients per serving: Calories: 83 kcal | Fat: 6g | Carbohydrates: 3g | Protein: 2g | Fiber: 1g

Ingredients

3 Tbsp. unsweetened almond milk (or a coconut milk)

3 Tbsp. sugar-free chocolate chips

3 ½ Tbsp. coconut oil melted

2 Tbsp. Lakanto Monkfruit (Powdered) Sweetener

2 eggs

1½ Tbsp. cocoa

1/3 cup of coconut flour

½ tsp. Vanilla

½ tsp. Salt

½ tsp. baking powder

½ Tbsp. Gelatin

¼ tsp. baking soda

Method

1.   Preheat the oven to 350 °F and spray the nonstick spray into a mini muffin pan. Only put aside.

2.   In a shallow mixing cup, combine the first 7 ingredients and whisk to combine, breaking up the clumps. To mix, add the next 4 ingredients and whisk well. Stir in the crisps of cookies. Scoop batter into any muffin cup with a cookie scoop (approximately 1 tbsp. of the batter). If needed, put 2-3 extra chocolate chips on every muffin and bake for about 10-12 minutes or until baked, at 350 °F . Do not bake in abundance. Before extracting, chill in the pot for 5-10 minutes and cool fully before enjoying.

17   Low Carb Dairy Free Coconut Cake

Servings: 12 | **Time**: 45 mins | **Difficulty**: Easy

Nutrients per serving: Calories: 257 kcal | Fat: 23g | Carbohydrates: 7g | Protein: 7g | Fiber: 3g

Ingredients

For the Cake:

6 eggs room temperature

2 cup almond flour

3 tsp. baking powder

1 Tsp. vanilla extract

1/2 tsp. salt

1/2 tsp. coconut extract

1/3 cup coconut oil melted

1/3 cup coconut cream

1/4 cup coconut flour

3/4 cup Lakanto Monkfruit Sweetener

For the Coconut Glaze:

Garnish: Whipped Coconut Cream

1/2 cup coconut cream

1/2 Tbsp. Lakanto Monkfruit Sweetener

1/4 tsp. coconut extract

Method

1.   Preheat the oven to 350 °F and oiled a 9-inch circular inch cake pan with parchment on the sides. Only put aside.

2.   Beat the 6 eggs in a medium-high to the stand mixer's high mixing bowl for 3-4 minutes. You need them to almost double volume and to be fluffy and light. Meanwhile, in a small bowl, combine the next five ingredients and mix to combine.

3.   Include the eggs' dry ingredients until the eggs are fluffy and light and doubled in volume, and blend well to mixed. Now, apply the extracts, coconut milk, molten coconut oil, and mix one more time to scrap the bowl's sides and ensure that it is well blended.

4.   Give the batter one last swirl to guarantee that you have the batter from the bottom of the bowl. Pour the batter into the prepared cake pan and bake for 25-30 minutes at 350 or until checked by a tester. Do not bake in excess.

5.   Combine the coconut glaze ingredients in a microwave-safe mixing cup while the cake is baking. Heat at intervals of 30 seconds, swirling each time until the sweetener has fully dissolved.   That can also be accomplished in a tiny saucepan over medium-low heat on the stovetop.

6.   Let it rest and cool for about 5-10 minutes until the cake is finished. Then pour over the warm cake with the coconut glaze. Before turning it out, cool the cake in a pan completely. Cut and serve with a whipped coconut cream garnish.

18   Buttered Rum Cake

Servings: 15 | **Time:** 1 hr | **Difficulty:** Easy

Nutrients per serving: Calories: 208 kcal | Fat: 16g | Carbohydrates: 5g | Protein: 5g | Fiber: 2g

Ingredients

For the Cake:

8 eggs

7 Tbsp. butter salted

3/4 cup coconut flour

2/3 cup Lakanto Golden Monkfruit Sweetener

2 tsp. baking powder

1/2 tsp salt

1 tsp. vanilla extract

1 tsp. baking soda

1 cup almond flour

¼ cup dark rum

¼ cup + 2 Tbsp sour cream

For the Glaze:

¼ cup of Lakanto Golden Monkfruit Sweetener

2 tbsp water

3 tbsp dark rum 4 tbsp butter

Method

1.   Preheat the oven to 350°F. Oil or spray an 8-9' loaf pan and line the bundt pan with parchment either spray and prepare it. Melt butter in a small skillet over low-medium heat, like a 3-4 environment. Continue to cook the butter for around 7-10 minutes, stirring until the butter is nutty and browned. The caramel color can be the solids in the butter. Remove from the heat and cool off.

2.   Whip eggs until light, foamy three times in volume using the stand mixer and a whisk. This can also be achieved using a handheld mixer, but to avoid splatter, use a big cup.

3.   Turn to paddle attachment while using a stand mixer. Add sweetener and blend. Add almond and coconut flour, cinnamon, baking powder, and baking soda to the egg mixture and mix until mixed at low pressure, rubbing downsides for at least once. Add the butter with sour cream, vanilla and browned butter, and rum and mix until combined. Spoon the batter uniformly into the pan and smooth the top. Bake for 35-40

minutes with a bundt at 350 °F or 45 minutes to an hour. Halfway through baking and partially covered with foil to avoid browning. The baking period would be marginally shorter if you have a 9' loaf pan, so keep an eye that it starting at 30 minutes.

4.   Please prepare the glaze while the cake is baking. Mix all the ingredients for a glaze in the same pan you used to brown the butter. Over medium pressure, bring the mixture to a boil and simmer for 2-3 minutes.

5.   Take it out of the oven and spread the glaze uniformly over the warm cake until the cake is finished. In the dish, cool the cake. The day before it's served, this cake is better made. Switch out onto your cake stand or tray of choice. Use the parchment to remove the loaf from a pan and slice to life if you cooked it in a loaf pan. Serve and eat with a coffee cup with a dollop of delivered milk. The cake can be stored at room temperature.

19 Chocolate Sour Cream Cake with Cream Cheese Frosting

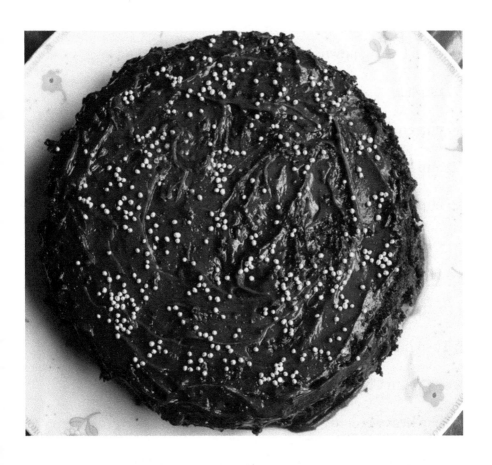

Servings: 12 | **Time:** 35 mins | **Difficulty:** Easy

Nutrients per serving: Calories: 226 kcal | Fat: 20g | Carbohydrates: 3g | Protein: 6.2g | Fiber: 2g

Ingredients

8 eggs

1/3 cup Pyure

1 tsp vanilla

1 ½ tsp baking powder

½ tsp salt

½ cup coconut flour

½ cup of butter melted

½ cup almond flour

¼ cup sour cream

¼ cup dutch cocoa (I use Rodelle Baking Cocoa) Cream Cheese Frosting

3 Tbsp butter softened

3 oz Cream Cheese softened

1 Tbsp heavy cream

½ tsp vanilla (I use Rodelle Pure Vanilla Extract)

½ cup powdered Lakanto Sweetener

Method

1.   Preheat the oven to 325°C. Spray or oil a 9-inch circular cake pan put it aside, and line the   base with parchment.

2.   Beat the 8 eggs in a medium-high to the stand mixer's high mixing bowl for 3-4 minutes. Double in volume and to be soft and bright. Meanwhile, in a small bowl, combine the next Six dry ingredients and mix to combine.

3.   Add dry ingredients in the eggs until the eggs are fluffy and doubled in volume and blend well. Now apply the sour cream, molten butter, and vanilla, then mix one more time to make sure it is mixed properly, rubbing the bowl's downsides.

4.   Give the batter one last swirl to guarantee that you have the batter from the base of the bowl. Pour the batter into the lined pan and bake for 25-30 minutes at 325 or until checked by a tester. Oh, don't overbake. Before turning it out, cool the cake in a pan completely.

5.   To make the frosting: In a medium dish, combine the cream cheese and the butter and beat until smooth with the handheld blender. Apply the vanilla, milk, and sweetener and stir until smooth and all the ingredients are mixed.

6.   Turn the cake out on a cake tray or platter until it's cold. Top and enjoy the frosting

20 Coconut Key Lime Bars

Servings: 16 | **Time**: 30 mins | **Difficulty:** Easy

Nutrients per serving: Calories: 216 kcal | Fat: 20g | Carbohydrates: 4g | Protein: 5g | Fiber: 1g

Ingredients

For the crust:

7 Tbsp salted butter melted

2 tsp lime zest

2 cups almond flour

1/3 cup Lakanto Golden Monkfruit Sweetener or your

1:1 Sweetener of Choice

½ cup shredded unsweetened coconut

¼ tsp. salt For the filling:

1/3 cup + 2Tbsp Lakanto Monkfruit (Golden) Sweetener

¼ cup key lime juice

2 whole eggs

5 egg yolks

5 Tbsp. butter cut into small pieces

1 Tbsp. coconut oil

1 Tbsp. powdered gelatin

½ tsp. vanilla extract

¼ tsp. coconut extract

Method

1.   To 350 °F, preheat the oven. Spray a 9 to 9 square pan with the parchment and line it. Lift the bars from the pan to remove them if you make the parchment strips, which are 9 inches wide enough to go up two on foot.

2.   Combine the first 5 ingredients for the crust in a mixing bowl and blend well to combine. To achieve a crumbly texture, apply the melted butter and blend. Uniformly press this mixture onto the bottom of a lined tray. Made sure you have decent corners and margins.Bake about 10-12 minutes or until the crust begins to light golden brown at 350 °F. Take it out of the oven and set it aside.

3.   Blend the main lime juice, eggs, sweetener, and yolks in a saucepan and whisk well to merge. To the pan, apply the butter and coconut oil. Turn the heat to low-medium (3-4 attitude) and start heating the mixture, stirring continuously. The butter will continue to melt as the mixture heats, stirring constantly. All the

butter will melt after about 5 minutes, and the filling will then start thickening. Keep stirring, but do not boil. Remove from the heat until the filling is thickened to a loose pudding. Sprinkle the gelatin generously over the surface of the filling and stir to mix instantly. Stir the extracts in.

4.   Pour the filling of lime uniformly over the top of a crust. Bake for 10-12 minutes at 350 or until set. Until cutting, cool properly. Use the overhanging parchment for lifting the bars from the pan until it is cool. To end up with 16 bars, make 4 even cuts horizontally and vertically.

21 Keto Lemon Pound Cake with Blueberries

Servings: 12 | **Time**: 30 mins | **Difficulty**: Easy

Nutrients per serving: Calories: 239 kcal | Fat: 21g | Carbohydrates: 7g | Protein: 8g | Fiber: 3g

Ingredients

11/4 cup almond flour

3/4 cup Lakanto Monkfruit Sweetener or any equivalent sweetener of choice

1/4 cup butter softened

1/2 Tsp. salt

1/2 cup fresh blueberries

4 oz cream cheese softened Zest of

2 lemons

4 eggs room temperature

1 Tsp. vanilla extract

1 Tbsp. coconut flour

1 Tsp. baking powder

2 tsp confectioners sweetener

Method

1.   Preheat a 350-degree oven and oil a 9-5-inch loaf pan. Only put aside,

2.   Combine the almond flour, baking powder, coconut flour, and salt in a medium dish.

3.   Cream butter with sweetener in a mixing bowl until fluffy and smooth. Apply the cream cheese and blend to ensure no lumps.

4.   Add the eggs one at a time to the butter mixture, combining thoroughly after each addition: Include vanilla and zest.

5.   For butter and eggs, add dry ingredients to the mixture. Mix well before blended well. Fold in the blueberries, taking care not to break them down. You should toss the blueberries with 2 tsp whether you have a powdered swerve or some other sweetener, which will make the cake's bottom to sink.

6.   Load the batter into a 9-5 inch oiled loaf bowl. For 40-45 minutes, bake. After 30 minutes, start testing for density.

7.   Remove from the oven and leave to cool for 25 minutes, then cool fully on the rack before slicing.

22   Mini Orange Cranberry Cheesecake

Servings: 12 | **Time**: 35 mins | **Difficulty**: Easy

Nutrients per serving: Calories: 144 kcal | Fat: 8g | Carbohydrates: 8g | Protein: 8g | Fiber: 2g

Ingredients

For the Crust:

Pinch salt

3 Tbsp salted butter melted

2 Tbsp Lakanto Monkfruit (Classic) Sweetener

1 cup almond flour

¼ tsp. cinnamon

For the Filling:

2/3 cup Lakanto Monkfruit (Classic) Sweetener

2 eggs

16 oz. packages cream cheese softened

1 tsp. vanilla

½ tsp. fresh orange zest

For the Cranberry Compote:

1 cup of water

1/2 cup Lakanto Gold Monkfruit Sweetener

1/8 tsp. ground clove

12 oz. bag fresh cranberries

2 Tbsp. Pyure Organic Stevia Blend

3-4 pieces orange peel inch wide by 4 inches long

Pinch salt

Method

1.   Put all the ingredients in the compote in a medium saucepan on medium heat. Simmer for 10-12 minutes before the cranberries burst and the sauce thickens. Remove from the heat and encourage to stay for thirty minutes. Remove the peel, drain into the serving bowl, and cool before serving time. In a zip-top bag or plastic ware, you can freeze as well. To serve, thaw in the refrigerator.

2.   Preheat the oven to 350 °F and use liners to cover a muffin tray. Mix the ingredients for a crust in a medium mixing

bowl and blend until combined and crumbly. Place roughly 1 Tbsp. In each muffin cup, blend the crust mixture and press it into each cup's rim. Only put aside.

3.   Mix the ingredients for filling in a medium mixing bowl and blend with a hand mixer. Between the 12 muffin cups, split the filling. Bake for 15-20 minutes at 350 °F or until set. Don't bake too much. Cool at room temperature and prepare until served in the fridge.

4.   Remove the cooled cheesecake wrapper and put it on the counter. Spoon the top of each cheesecake with about two Tbsp. of cranberry compote and enjoy.

23 Keto Double Fudge Cookies

Servings: 12 | **Time:** 15 mins | **Difficulty**: Easy

Nutrients per serving: Calories: 63 kcal | Fat: 5g | Carbohydrates: 3g | Protein: 2g | Fiber: 1g

Ingredients

¼ cup creamy almond butter

½ cup Lily's Chocolate Chips

½ cup Rodelle Gourmet Baking Cocoa

½ tsp. Baking powder

½ tsp. salt

1 Tbsp. coconut flour

1 tsp. Rodelle Vanilla Extract

1/3 cup + 1 Tbsp. Lakanto Monkfruit (Powdered) Sweetener

2 eggs

2 Tbsp. salted butter softened

Method

1.   Preheat the oven to 350 °F and use parchment to cover a sheet plate. Mix the butter and the almond butter in a medium bowl until thoroughly integrated. Include the vanilla and eggs and combine until smooth.

2.   The next Five ingredients are added and blend properly. Stir in the crisps of cookies. Use a cookie scoop to release flour on the lined sheet pan about 2 inches apart. Slightly flatten those cookies with wet fingertips. They won't scatter much throughout the baking process.

3.   Bake for Six minutes for the fudgy texture or the less fudgy texture for 7 minutes. Don't bake too much. Let it cool on the sheet pan for 2-3 minutes, then remove to cool fully. They will set up as the cookies cool, so be careful.

24 Low Carb Acai Berry Bowl

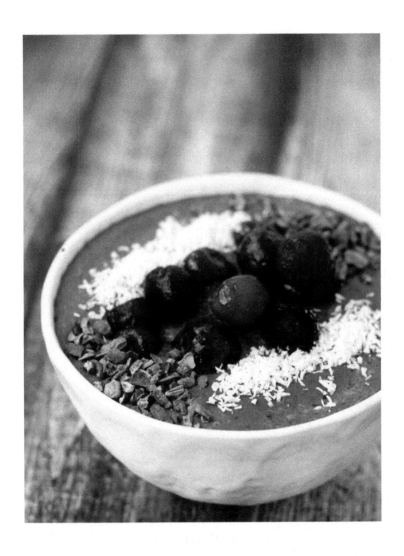

Servings: 1 | **Time:** 5 mins | **Difficulty:** Easy

Nutrients per serving: Calories: 202 kcal | Fat: 13g | Carbohydrates: 18g | Protein: 2g | Fiber: 10g

Ingredients

Acai Berry Base

4 strawberries

3 tsp acai powder

1 tsp Pyure Organic Stevia Blend

Pinch of Himalayan Salt

1/3 cup avocado

1/3 cup unsweetened almond milk

1/4 cup blueberries

Garnishes / Topping Optional

blueberries or raspberries chia seeds

low carb granola pecans

shaved coconut sliced strawberries

Method

1.   Combine all the Acai Berry base ingredients in a high-speed blender and then blend for 10 seconds or until smooth and fluffy.

2.   Pour into a little mug, garnish, and enjoy your morning as desired.

25   Keto Fudge Ribbon Cake

Servings: 16 | **Time:** 1 hr | **Difficulty:** Easy

Nutrients per serving: Calories: 258 kcal | Fat: 23g | Carbohydrates: 8g | Protein: 7g | Fiber: 4g

Ingredients

½ cup avocado oil

½ cup coconut flour

½ tsp salt

1 ½ cup almond flour

1 ½ tsp baking powder

1 cup Lakanto Golden Monkfruit Sweetener (we use Lakanto and Highkey Allulose)

1 tsp vanilla

1 tsp. baking soda

1/2 cup cocoa

1/2 cup full-fat sour cream

6 eggs

Cream Cheese Frosting:

1 tsp. vanilla

2 eggs

2 Tbsp. butter softened

2 Tbsp. coconut flour

6 Tbsp. powdered Lakanto Sweetener

8 oz. cream cheese softened

Method

1.   Preheat the oven to 350°C. Oiled a 10 cup tray and sprinkle with cocoa thoroughly. By tapping the pan on the sink, extract any extra cocoa. Oil the inside, line the bottom layer and sides with parchment while using loaf pans, and set them aside.

2.   Beat the 6 eggs in a medium-high to the high mixing bowl of a stand mixer for 2-3 minutes, until light and fluffy. In the meantime, in a tiny cup, combine the next Seven dry ingredients and combine them.

3.   Add the eggs' dry ingredients until the eggs become light and fluffy and doubled in volume and blend well to mixed. Now apply oil, sour cream, and vanilla and mix one more time to scrape down the bowl's sides to ensure that it is well mixed and pour the batter into the bowl.

4. Mix the cream cheese, butter, vanilla, powdered sweetener, coconut flour, and eggs in a separate cup, and beat until well mixed. Pour the combination of cream cheese generously on the chocolate batter.

5. For 45-50 minutes, bake at 350. Cool the cake in a pan for 10-15 minutes to cool entirely on a rack or plate before turning out. Cold top once as needed and serve. Store at room temperature up to 3 days.

Snack

26   Golden Potato Croquettes

Servings: 4 | **Time:** 5 mins | **Difficulty**: Easy

Nutrients per serving: Calories: 331 kcal | Fat: 30g | Carbohydrates: 2g | Protein: 13g | Fiber: 0g

Ingredients

2 oz. butter

8 oz. (2 cups) cheddar cheese or provolone cheese, in slices

Method

1.   On the large cutting board, put the cheese slices.

2.   Cut the butter with the cheese slicer or us1e a knife to cut tiny bits.

3.   Use butter to coat every cheese slice and roll-up. Now Serve as snacks.

27   Sugar-Free Keto Low Carb Granola Bars

Servings: 12 | **Time**: 40 mins | **Difficulty:** Easy

Nutrients per serving: Calories: 194 kcal | Fat: 17.4g | Carbohydrates: 8.3g | Protein: 5.5g | Fiber: 4.6g

Ingredients

4 Tbsp Monkfruit

3/4 tsp Sea salt

2 Tbsp Almond butter

1/4 cup Stevia chocolate chips (sweetened and dairy-free)

1 Tbsp Coconut oil

1 large egg

1 cup coconut flakes (Unsweetened and tightly packed (65g))

1 Cup Slivered almonds (85g)

1 Cup Raw almonds, Chopped (140g)

Method

1.   1.Heat your oven up to 375 °F and line parchment paper with an 8x8 inch pan. Leave some hanging on the sides to be used later as a handle.

2.   On 3 separate small baking sheets, put the sliced almonds, coconut flakes, and slivered almonds. Bake until toasted and golden colored. It takes 2-4 minutes for the coconut, about 3-5 minutes for the slivered almonds, and about 7-12 minutes for the chopped almonds. Please enable it to cool fully. Also, decrease the temperature of the oven to 350.

3.   Whisk the egg and the monk fruit in a large bowl together.

4.   Melt the almond butter and the coconut oil in a separate, tight, microwave-safe bowl until smooth, for about 30 seconds. Whisk in the combination of eggs when well mixed.

5.   Put in all the almonds, salt, and coconut and mix until well mixed. Whisk in the chocolate chips at last.

6.   Put a few muscles into it because then they stay together; you have to pack these in.

7.   Cook until the top seems set, at 350 °F for about 15 minutes. Let it cool fully in the pan to room temperature. Slice and DEVOUR when cold

28 Sauteed Broccolini

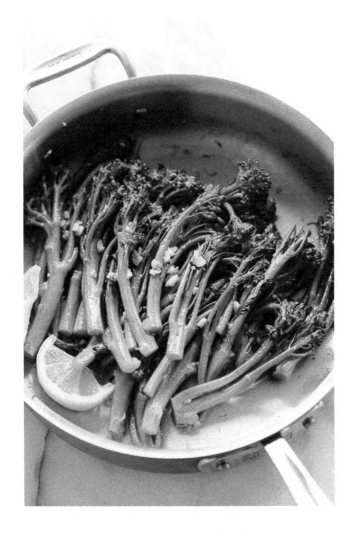

Servings: 4 | **Time:** 20 mins | **Difficulty**: Easy

Nutrients per serving: Calories: 40 kcal | Fat: 3.4g | Carbohydrates: 1g | Protein: 1g | Fiber: 1g

Ingredients

1/2 Cup Water

1/2 tsp Garlic, diced

1 Lb Broccolini

1 Tbsp Olive oil Salt

Method

1.   Cut off the broccolini's stalky ends and drop some flowers.

2.   Place the broccolini with the water in a vast, high-sided skillet and move to medium heat. Cover and cook until a broccolini is light green and stirring regularly, around 8-10 mins.

3.   Uncover and cook for about 1-2 minutes before the water dries.

4.   Push the broccolini aside and add the garlic and oil. Stir and cook together until the broccolini is brown and burnt a little.

5.   Season with salt and DEVOUR to perfection.

29 Marinated Olives

Servings: 6 | **Time:** 20 mins | **Difficulty**: Easy

Nutrients per serving: Calories: 161 kcal | Fat: 16.31g | Carbohydrates: 4.96g | Protein: 0.28g | Fiber: 0.5g

Ingredients

3 tbsp olive oil

2 tsp chopped fresh parsley (basil or tarragon)

1-2 tbsp red wine vinegar (or lemon juice)

1/4 tsp salt

1/4 tsp red pepper flakes

1 tsp whole fennel seeds

1 tsp chopped fresh rosemary (or thyme)

1 medium garlic clove, minced

1 cup medium pitted green olives (6 oz)

1 cup medium pitted black olives (6 oz)

Method

1.   In a small saucepan on medium-low heat, heat the fennel seeds until fragrant.

2.   Switch the fire to medium and add the flakes of olive oil, vinegar, garlic, rosemary (or thyme), and red pepper. Heat until fragrant with the oil, around 8 minutes.

3.   Pour the olives over them and stir. Add salt and parsley, swirling to mix. Serve instantly, then let marinate for an excellent taste for about 2 hours.

4.   Alternately, in a mortar with the pestle, smash the fennel seeds. Garlic is then added and worked into a paste. For the next seven ingredients, stir in. For the marinade, toss the olives. For the most pleasing taste, marinate for many hours.

5.   STORE: Put in an airtight jar or a film-coated bowl and can refrigerate for one week.

30   Keto Snickerdoodles

Servings: 8 | **Time:** 10 mins | **Difficulty**: Easy

Nutrients per serving: Calories: 57 kcal | Fat: 5.2g | Carbohydrates: 8.6g | Protein: 1.2g | Fiber: 1g

Ingredients

0.63 cups Almond Flour (125g)

2 Tbsp Coconut flour, packed (28g)

0.5 tsp Vanilla

0.5 Egg

0.5 tsp Cream of tartar

0.5 tsp Cinnamon

0.13 tsp Salt

0.25 cup + 1 Tbsp Swerve, divided

0.25 tsp Xantham gum (do not omit)

2.5 Tbsp Unsalted Butter, softened to room temperature (70g)

Method

1.   Heat the oven to 350 °F. Place parchment paper on a baking sheet.

2.   Mix Cream Butter and 1/2 cup swerve until smooth with the electric hand mixer. Include the egg and vanilla, then beat until well mixed.

3.   Apply all the remaining ingredients, except cinnamon and the remainder of Swerve, and stir until combined.

4.   On a small pan, mix the cinnamon and swerve. Roll the dough into balls and measure 1 Tbsp, and put on the cookie sheet.

5.   Slightly press the 1/3 inch thick balls and bake for 12-13 minutes before the edges start to feel set. And let pan fully cool down and DEVOUR.

31   Roasted Air Fryer Cauliflower

Servings: 4 | **Time**: 25 mins | **Difficulty:** Easy

Nutrients per serving: Calories: 41 kcal | Fat: 2.4g | Carbohydrates: 4.4g | Protein: 1.7g | Fiber: 2.1g

Ingredients

2 tsp Olive oil

3/4 Lb Cauliflower, cut into florets

Sea salt

Method

1.   In a wide cup, put cauliflower florets and drizzle with the oil, tossing them to cover. Then, sprinkle with salt generously.

2.   Place in a single layer in the air fryer's mesh basket and cook at 400 F until golden brown and fork-tender, around 17-22 minutes.

32 Salt And Pepita Hard Boiled Egg Snack

Servings: 8 | **Time:** 35 mins | **Difficulty:** Easy

Nutrients per serving: Calories: 94.5 kcal | Fat: 6.7g | Carbohydrates: 0.7g | Protein: 7.7g | Fiber: 0.3g

Ingredients

8 large Eggs

1 tsp Sea Salt

1/4-1/2 tsp Black Pepper (depending on you, how peppery you like your eggs)

1/4 cup Pepitas

Method

1.   Preheat to 400°F in your oven.

2.   Place the eggs in the thin layer in a huge jar. Cover them and put them to a boil on high heat with 2 inches of water. Switch off the heat (but do not remove the pot from), cover and pot until they hit a rolling boil, and leave around 10-12 minutes.

Pour the water and cover it with cold water, and let it stand for 10 minutes.

3.   Place the pepitas over a small baking sheet while the eggs become fried and bake until softly golden brown, around 5-7 minutes.

4.   Switch the toasted pepitas, pepper, and salt to the small food processor or the spice grinder and pulse until these broken down, but there are some small bits of texture.

5.   By dipping into the mixture of pepitas, peel the eggs and DEVOUR

33 Crispy Air Fryer Brussels Sprouts

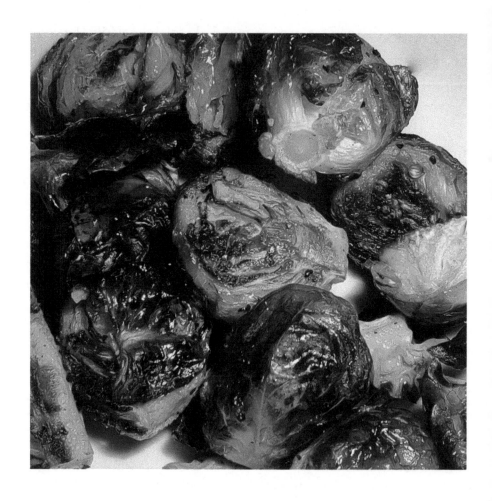

Servings: 4 | **Time:** 35 mins | **Difficulty**: Easy

Nutrients per serving: Calories: 78.2 kcal | Fat: 3.7g | Carbohydrates: 10.1g | Protein: 3.8g | Fiber: 4.3g

Ingredients

Sea salt

1 Tbsp Olive oil

1 Lb Brussels sprouts

Method

1.   Heat your fryer in the air to 350 F

2.   Trim the ends of the sprouts in Brussels, cut the leaves and not look good. After trimming, you can end up with around 3/4 lb of the Brussels sprouts,

3.   Place the Brussels in a bowl and toss with salt and olive oil. Remove and set aside any singular leaves for later.

4.   Put the Brussels inside your air fryer's mesh basket and cook for about 12 minutes. Next, shake the basket, then cook for a further 10-12 minutes before you're done with the Brussels look. Put the singular leaves in the air fryer at this stage and cook for 2 to 3 minutes until crispy.

34   Sugar-Free Keto No Bake Cookies

Servings: 12 | **Time:** 10 mins | **Difficulty**: Easy

Nutrients per serving: Calories: 156.4 kcal | Fat: 14.4g | Carbohydrates: 5.7g | Protein: 3.8g | Fiber: 2.8g

Ingredients

pinch of Salt

6 tbsp Almond Butter (the no-stir kind)

2 tbsp of Unsalted Butter (or dairy-free butter)

2 tbsp of Sugar-Free Chocolate Chips (or dairy-free)

2 1/2 tbsp Monkfruit Sweetener

1/2 cup Unsweetened Coconut Flakes

1 1/4 cups Almond Flour, (125g)

Method

1.   Melt the almond butter & butter until they become smooth and creamy, around 1 minute, in a big, microwave-safe dish.

2.	Whisk until it is absorbed in the monk fruit. Then stir in almond flour, the flakes of coconut, and salt.

3.	To cool, put the bowl in the fridge for 15 minutes.

4.	Whisk in the chocolate chips until cooled.

5.	Roll into balls of 1 1/2 Tbsp and put on a cookie sheet lined with parchment paper. Slightly push out, to around 1/2 inch thick.

6.	For at least an hour, cover and refrigerate.

35 Grilled Avocados With Feta Tahini Sauce

Servings: 6 | **Time:** 10 mins | **Difficulty**: Easy

Nutrients per serving: Calories: 199 kcal | Fat: 18.1g | Carbohydrates: 9.4g | Protein: 3.2g | Fiber: 6.2g

Ingredients

1 Garlic clove

2 tsp Fresh lemon juice

2 tsp Olive oil

3 Large Fresh Avocados

Salt

For The Sauce:

1/4 cup Feta cheese, crumbled (37g)

1 1/2 Tbsp Tahini

1/2 - 1 Tbsp Reduced-sodium chicken broth (depending on how thick you like your sauce)

4 tsp Fresh lemon juice

1 tsp Honey Pinch of salt

Method

1.   Preheat to medium-high heat on your barbecue.

2.   Cut the avocados in half, and the seeds are removed. Peel a clove of garlic and take the top off. Everywhere on the cut side of avocado, rub the cut portion of the garlic.

3.   In a shallow bowl, mix the olive oil and the lemon juice and spray over the avocados. Sprinkle salt on it.

4.   Place the cut side down over the grill and cook for around 5-6 minutes before excellent grill marks are created.

5.   Place the feta in the small microwave-safe bowl, then microwave it for about 10-15 seconds before cooking and softening, using a small food processor to mix all the sauce ingredients. To make sure it gets clean and creamy, you'll need to pause, scrape down each side, and then resume blending again—season with salt to taste.

6.   Divide the sauce among the avocados, squeeze with the fresh lemon juice (not mandatory) and scoop to DEVOUR straight from the pod.

Beverages

36 McKeto Strawberry Milkshake

Servings: 1 | **Time:** 5 mins | **Difficulty:** Easy

Nutrients per serving: Calories: 368 kcal | Fat: 38.85g | Carbohydrates: 2.42g | Protein: 1.69g | Fiber: 1.28g

Ingredients

1/4 Cup Heavy Cream

1/4 Tsp. Xanthan Gum

3/4 Cup Coconut Milk

7 Ice Cubes

1 Tbsp. MCT Oil

2 Tbsps. Strawberry Torani, Sugar-Free

Method

1.   Combine all the ingredients in a blender and mix until a smooth consistency is attained.

2.   Decant into the serving glass and enjoy.

37 Keto Blueberry Cheesecake Smoothie

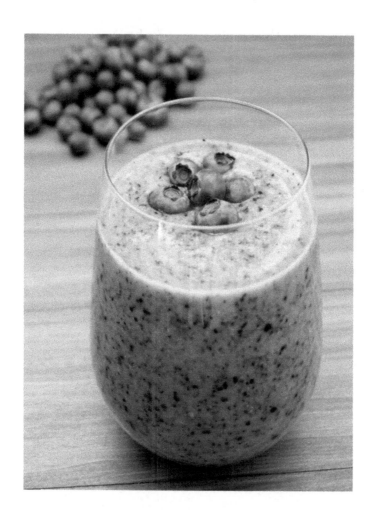

Servings: 1 | **Time:** 5 mins | **Difficulty**: Easy

Nutrients per serving: Calories: 311 kcal | Fat: 27g | Carbohydrates: 9g | Protein: 5.5g | Fiber: 2.5g

Ingredients

1/2 Cup Cream Cheese

2 Tbsps. Heavy Cream

1 Cup Almond Milk, Unsweetened

1 Tsp. Cinnamon, Ground

1/2 Cup Blueberries

6 Drops Stevia

1/2 Tsp. Vanilla Extract

Method

1.   Combine all the ingredients in a blender and mix until a smooth consistency is attained.

2.   Decant into the serving glass and enjoy.

38   Keto Tropical Smoothie

Servings: 2 | **Time:** 5 mins | **Difficulty:** Easy

Nutrients per serving: Calories: 355.75 kcal | Fat: 32.63g | Carbohydrates: 4.41g | Protein: 4.4g | Fiber: 3g

Ingredients

1 Tbsp. MCT Oil

1/2 Tsp. Mango Extract

7 Ice Cubes

2 Tbsps. Golden Flaxseed Meal

1/4 Tsp. Blueberry Extract

3/4 Cup Coconut Milk, Unsweetened

1/4 Tsp. Banana Extract

1/4 Cup Sour Cream

20 Drops Liquid Stevia

Method

1.   Combine all the ingredients in a blender and mix until a smooth consistency is attained. Let it sit for a few minutes and allow the flax meal to absorb moisture.

2.   Decant into the serving glasses and enjoy.

39   Keto Kale & Coconut Shake

Servings: 1 | **Time:** 5 mins | **Difficulty:** Easy

Nutrients per serving: Calories: 660 kcal | Fat: 60g | Carbohydrates: 7g | Protein: 13g | Fiber: 7g

Ingredients

4 Cups Kale, Chopped

1/2 Cup Coconut Milk

1 Cup Almond Milk, Unsweetened

1/4 Cup Coconut, Unsweetened & Ground

1 Cup Ice

1/4 Tsp. Kosher Salt

1Tbsp. Fresh Ginger, Peeled (Optional)

Method

1.   Combine all the ingredients in a blender and mix until a smooth consistency is attained.

2.   Decant into the serving glass and enjoy.

40 Savory Cucumber Herb Sangria

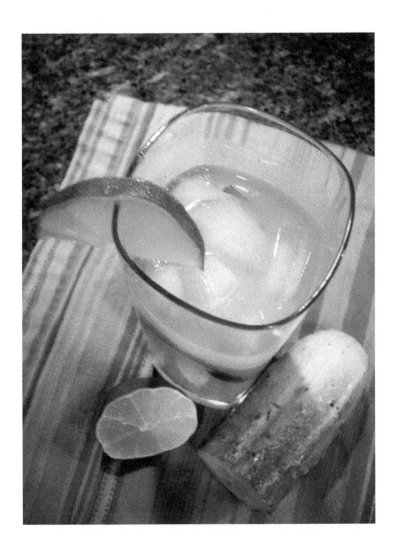

Servings: 2-4 | **Time:** 5 mins | **Difficulty**: Easy

Nutrients per serving: Calories: 660 kcal | Fat: 60g | Carbohydrates: 7g | Protein: 13g | Fiber: 7g

Ingredients

2 Cups Sparkling Water

3 Cups Dry White Wine

2 Cups Ice

3 Limes, Sliced

1 Green Cucumber, Sliced

1 Cup Basil Leaves, Fresh

2 Lemons, Sliced

1 Cup Mint Leaves, Fresh

Method

1.   Put all ingredients in a pitcher except wine, sparkling water, and ice. Stir well and press the lemon, lime, basil, mint, and cucumber a little to release their juices.

2.   Add the wine to it and stir well.

3.   Put it in the refrigerator and let it sit for about 20 minutes.

4.   Take out the pitcher and pour in the sparkling water and ice.

5.   Serve cold.

41 Sparkling Raspberry Limeade Mocktail

Servings: 2 | **Time:** 1 min | **Difficulty**: Easy

Nutrients per serving: Calories: 22 kcal | Fat: 0.2g | Carbohydrates: 5.5g | Protein: 0.5g | Fiber: 2.1g

Ingredients

1/2 Cup Raspberries, Unsweetened & Frozen

1 & 1/2 Cups Sparkling Raspberry Lemonade, Chilled

2 Tbsps. Lime Juice

1/8 Tsp. Vanilla Stevia

1/2 Cup Ice, Crushed

Method

1. Combine all the ingredients in a blender and mix until a smooth consistency is attained.

2. Decant into the serving glasses and enjoy.

42 Bailey's Irish Cream

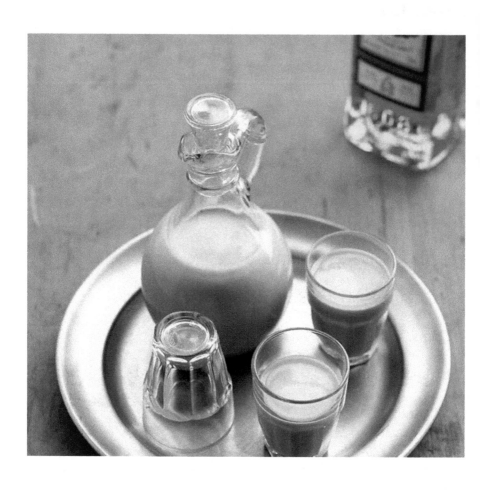

Servings: 12 | **Time:** 20 mins | **Difficulty:** Easy

Nutrients per serving: Calories: 200 kcal | Fat: 14g | Carbohydrates: 1g | Protein: 0g | Fiber: 0g

Ingredients

1/2 Tsp. Vanilla Extract

1 & 1/4 Cups Irish Whiskey

2 Cups Heavy Cream

1 Tbsp. Cocoa Powder

1/2 Tsp. Instant Espresso Powder

2/3 Cup Swerve

1 Tsp. Almond Extract

Method

1.   Take a saucepan and put cocoa, instant powder, sweetener, and cream in it. Heat it over medium-low flame and bring to a boil.

2.   Reduce heat to low and let it simmer for about 10 minutes.

3.   Take off the heat and add in the whiskey, almond, and vanilla extracts.

4.   Let cool and serve.

43 Low Carb Coffee Milkshake

Servings: 2 | **Time:** 1 min | **Difficulty**: Easy

Nutrients per serving: Calories: 345 kcal | Fat: 31.4g | Carbohydrates: 24g | Protein: 2.5g | Fiber: 18.2g

Ingredients

1 Tsp. Instant Espresso Powder

15 Drops Stevia

1 & 1/2 Cups Ice, Crushed

1 Cup Vanilla Ice Cream (Low Carb)

1/2 Cup Almond Milk

2 Tsps. Cocoa Powder (Optional)

2 Tbsps. Whipped Cream (Optional)

Method

1.   Combine all the ingredients in a blender and mix until a smooth consistency is attained.

2.   Decant into the serving glasses and put a dollop of whipped cream on top if you want.

44 Sugar-Free Strawberry Limeade

Servings: 8 | **Time:** 5 mins | **Difficulty:** Easy

Nutrients per serving: Calories: 16 kcal | Fat: 0.1g | Carbohydrates: 4.3g | Protein: 0.2g | Fiber: 1.5g

Ingredients

5 Cups Water

3/4 Cup Lime Juice, Fresh

1 & 1/2 Tsps. Stevia

1 & 1/2 Cups Strawberries, Sliced

Ice, To Taste

Method

1.   Combine all the ingredients in a blender and mix until a smooth consistency is attained.

2.   Decant into the serving glasses and enjoy.

45   Low-Carb Keto Shamrock Shake

Servings: 1 | **Time**: 2 mins | **Difficulty**: Easy

Nutrients per serving: Calories: 660 kcal | Fat: 60g | Carbohydrates: 7g | Protein: 13g | Fiber: 7g

Ingredients

1 Tsp. Spinach Powder

1 Cup Vanilla Ice Cream, Low Carb

1/3 Cup Coconut Or Almond Milk, Unsweetened

1/8 Tsp. Pure Mint Extract

Whipped Cream (Optional)

Method

1.   Combine all the ingredients in a blender and mix until a smooth consistency is attained.

2.   Decant into the serving glasses and put a dollop of whipped cream on top if you want.

46   Keto Smoothie With Almond Milk

Servings: 1 | **Time**: 5 mins | **Difficulty:** Easy

Nutrients per serving: Calories: 332 kcal | Fat: 28.5g | Carbohydrates: 15g | Protein: 10.2g | Fiber: 8.9g

Ingredients

1 Tbsp. Cocoa Powder, Unsweetened

2 Tbsps. Almond Butter

1 Cup Almond Milk

1/4 Cup Avocado

3 Tbsps. Monkfruit

1 Cup Ice, Crushed

Method

1.   Combine all the ingredients in a blender and mix until a smooth consistency is attained.

2.   Decant into the serving glass and enjoy.

47 Sparkling Grapefruit Frosé

Servings: 6 | **Time**: 5 mins | **Difficulty**: Easy

Nutrients per serving: Calories: 244 kcal | Fat: 0.1g | Carbohydrates: 29.1g | Protein: 1g | Fiber: 0.1g

Ingredients

1 Cup Ice

1 Cup Grapefruit Juice, Fresh

1/4 Cup Agave Nectar

1 & 1/2 Cups Rosé Wine For Garnish (Optional)

Grapefruit Wedges Mint Sprigs

Method

1.   Freeze rosé in a shallow dish overnight.

2.   Scrape it off the dish the next day and put in a blender with all other ingredients.

3.   Blend until a smooth consistency is attained.

4.   Decant into the serving glasses and garnish with mint sprigs and grapefruit wedges if you want.

48 Banana Oat Breakfast Smoothie

Servings: 2 | **Time:** 5 mins | **Difficulty**: Easy

Nutrients per serving: Calories: 210 kcal | Fat: 7.5g | Carbohydrates: 32.5g | Protein: 5.6g | Fiber: 4.8g

Ingredients

1 Banana

1/2 Cup Almond Milk

1 Tbsp. Flaxseed Meal

1/2 Cup Yogurt

1/2 Tsp. Cinnamon

1/3 Cup Rolled Oats

Method

1.   Combine all the ingredients in a blender and mix until a smooth consistency is attained.

2.   Decant into the serving glasses and enjoy.

49   Keto Mexican Chocolate Eggnog

Servings: 6 | **Time:** 15 mins | **Difficulty:** Easy

Nutrients per serving: Calories: 242 kcal | Fat: 23g | Carbohydrates: 4g | Protein: 7g | Fiber: 1g

Ingredients

1/4 Cup Whiskey Or Bourbon

1 & 1/2 Cups Almond Milk, Unsweetened

6 Eggs

1/4 Cup Cocoa Powder

1/2 Cup Monkfruit/Erythritol Blend

1 Cup Heavy Cream

1/2 Cup Whipped Cream

1 Tsp. Vanilla

1/2 Tsp. Cinnamon Powder

1/4 Tsp. Chili Powder

1/8 Tsp. Cayenne Pepper

1/8 Tsp. Nutmeg, Grated

1/8 Tsp. Salt

Method

1.	Combine all the ingredients in a blender except bourbon/whiskey, vanilla, and whipped cream. Blend it until a smooth consistency is attained.

2.	Then pour this mixture into a saucepan and heat it over a medium-low flame with constant stirring for about 8 minutes. Do not let it boil.

3.	Take off the heat, put the saucepan in a bowl full of ice, and stir the eggnog to cool it down.

4.	Add the bourbon/whiskey and vanilla in it and decant into a covered container.

5.	Refrigerate for about 4 hours and add in the whipped cream or top the eggnog with it.

6.	Serve and enjoy.

50   Keto Cranberry Hibiscus Margarita

Servings: 8 | **Time:** 20 mins | **Difficulty:** Easy

Nutrients per serving: Calories: 86 kcal | Fat: 1g | Carbohydrates: 6g | Protein: 1g | Fiber: 2g

Ingredients

2 & 1/2 Tbsps. Naval Orange Zest

1 & 1/2 Cups Cranberries, Fresh

1 Cup Tequila

5 Cup Water

3/4 Cups + 2 Tbsps. Monkfruit/Erythritol Blend

3 Tbsps. Lime Juice, Fresh

Ice

4 Hibiscus Tea Bags

Coarse Salt, For Glass's Rim

Method

1.   Take a saucepan and put the 1 cup water, 3/4 cup sweetener, orange zest, and cranberries in it. Heat it over medium flame and bring to boil, reduce heat, and let it simmer until it is thickened, for about 10- 15 minutes.

2.   Strain the cranberry gel and let cool.

3.   Boil the remaining 4 cups of water in a saucepan and put the hibiscus tea bags in it for five minutes.

4.   Take out the tea bags and add the 2 Tbsps. of sweetener in it. Mix well and set aside to cool down.

5.   Combine the cranberry gel, hibiscus tea, and all the remaining ingredients in a blender and blend well.

6.   Slightly wet the rim of cocktail glasses and line with salt, and pour the margarita in them.

Lightning Source UK Ltd.
Milton Keynes UK
UKHW020419070521
383233UK00001BA/72